The Easy And Affordable Vegetarian Cooking Guide

Easy, Affordable And Tasty Vegetarian Recipes For Everyone

Riley Bloom

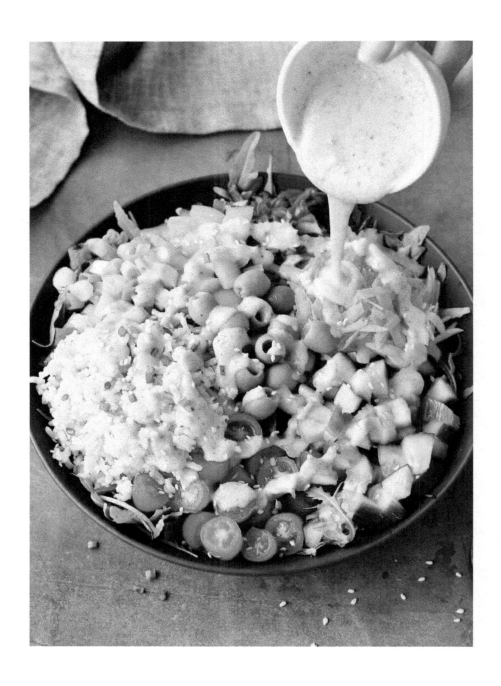

Table of contents

5

Vegetarian Alfredo Sauce

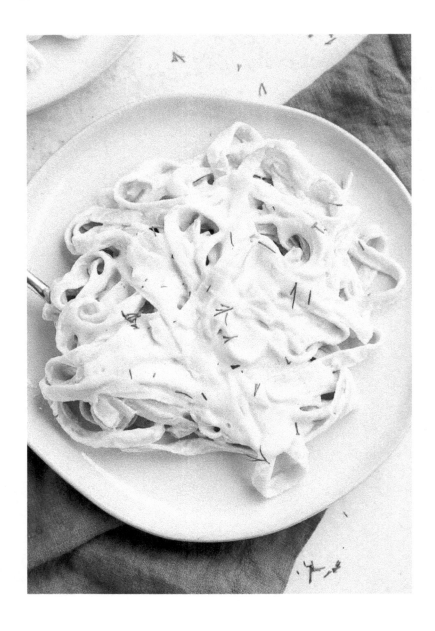

Ingredients

- 1/4 cup butter
- 3 cloves garlic, minced
- 2 cups cooked white beans, rinsed and drained
- 1 1/2 cups unsweetened almond milk
- Sea salt and pepper, to taste
- Parsley (optional)

Directions:

Melt the butter on low heat. Add the garlic and cook for 2 ½ minutes. Transfer to a food processor, add the beans and 1 cup of almond milk. Blend until smooth. Pour the sauce to the pan over low heat and season with salt and pepper. Add the parsley. Cook until warm.

Vegan Fajitas

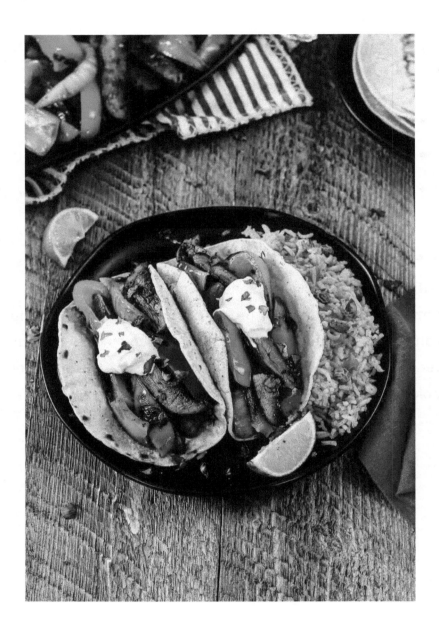

Ingredients

- 1 can Refried Beans (15oz)
- 1 can Lima Beans (15oz), drained and rinsed
- 1/4 cup Salsa
- 1 red Onion sliced into strips
- 1 Green Bell Pepper sliced into strips
- 2 Tbsp Lime Juice
- 2 tsp Fajita Spice Mix (see below)

<u>Tortillas Fajita Mix</u>

- 1 tbsp. Corn Starch
- 2 tsp Chili Powder
- 1 tsp Spanish Paprika
- 1 tsp honey
- 1/2 tsp Sea salt
- 1/2 teaspoon Onion Powder
- 1/2 teaspoon Garlic Powder
- 1/2 teaspoon Ground Cumin
- 1/8 teaspoon Cayenne Pepper

Directions:

Simmer salsa and refried beans until warm. Add and mix the fajita) mix ingredients in a small bowl and leave 2 tsp. behind. Sauté the onion, pepper, and 2 tsp of Spice Mix in water and lime juice Continue until liquid evaporates and vegetables start to brown Layer the beans in the middle of the tortilla. Layer with the stir-fried veggies and toppings. Roll it up and serve.

Mangoes Heirloom Tomatoes and Cucumber Salad

Ingredients:

- 1 cup of cubed mangoes

- 3 Heirloom tomatoes, halved lengthwise, seeded, and thinly sliced

- 1/4 white onion, peeled, halved lengthwise, and thinly sliced

- 1 large cucumber, halved lengthwise and thinly sliced

- 5 ounces cottage cheese, crumbled

Dressing

- ¼ cup extra-virgin olive oil

- 2 splashes white wine vinegar

- Coarse salt and black pepper

Directions:

Combine all of the dressing ingredients. Toss with the rest of the ingredients and combine well.

Black Grapes and Plum Tomato with Feta Cheese Salad

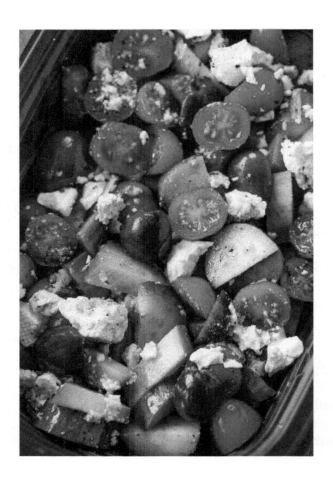

Ingredients:

- 12 pcs. black grapes

- 5 medium plum tomatoes, halved lengthwise, seeded, and thinly sliced

- 1/4 white onion, peeled, halved lengthwise, and thinly sliced

- 1 large cucumber, halved lengthwise and thinly sliced

- 2 ounces feta cheese, crumbled

- 2 ounces pepperjack cheese, shredded

Dressing

- ¼ cup extra-virgin olive oil

- 2 splashes white wine vinegar

- Coarse salt and black pepper

Directions:

Combine all of the dressing ingredients. Toss with the rest of the ingredients and combine well.

Napa Cabbage and Tomatillo with Pecorino Romano Salad

Ingredients:

- 1/2 medium Napa cabbage, sliced thinly
- 10 Tomatillos, halved lengthwise, seeded, and thinly sliced
- 1/4 white onion, peeled, halved lengthwise, and thinly sliced
- 1 large cucumber, halved lengthwise and thinly sliced
- 5 ounces pecorino romano cheese, shredded

Dressing

- ¼ cup extra-virgin olive oil
- 2 splashes white wine vinegar
- Coarse salt and black pepper

Directions:

Combine all of the dressing ingredients. Toss with the rest of the ingredients and combine well.

Pineapple Tomato & Cucumber Salad

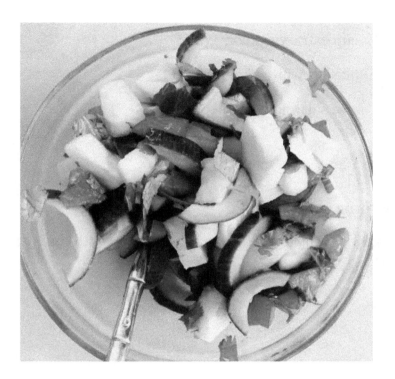

Ingredients:

- 1 cup canned pineapple bits

- 5 medium plum tomatoes, halved lengthwise, seeded, and thinly sliced

- 1/4 white onion, peeled, halved lengthwise, and thinly sliced

- 1 large cucumber, halved lengthwise and thinly sliced

17

- 5 ounces pecorino romano cheese, shredded

Dressing

- ¼ cup extra-virgin olive oil
- 2 splashes white wine vinegar
- Coarse salt and black pepper

Directions:

Combine all of the dressing ingredients. Toss with the rest of the ingredients and combine well.

Cherries Tomatoes and Onion Salad

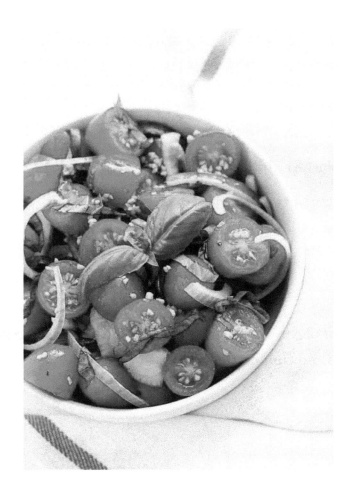

Ingredients:

- 1/4 cup cherries

- 3 Heirloom tomatoes, halved lengthwise, seeded, and thinly sliced

- 1/4 white onion, peeled, halved lengthwise, and thinly sliced
- 1 large Zucchini halved lengthwise, thinly sliced and blanched

Dressing

- ¼ cup extra-virgin olive oil
- 2 splashes white wine vinegar
- Coarse salt and black pepper

Directions:

Combine all of the dressing ingredients. Toss with the rest of the ingredients and combine well.

Tomatillo Corn and Cheddar Cheese Salad

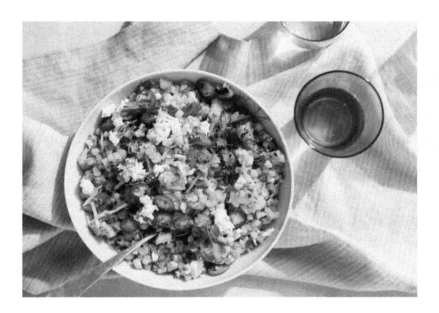

Ingredients:

- 10 Tomatillos, halved lengthwise, seeded, and thinly sliced

- 1/2 cup canned corn

- 1 large cucumber, halved lengthwise and thinly sliced

- 5 ounces cheddar cheese , shredded

<u>Dressing</u>

- ¼ cup extra-virgin olive oil

- 2 tbsp. apple cider vinegar

- Coarse salt and black pepper

Directions:

Combine all of the dressing ingredients. Toss with the rest of the ingredients and combine well.

Water Chestnuts Red Cabbage and Artichoke Salad

Ingredients:

- 1/2 cup canned water chestnuts

- 1/2 medium red cabbage, sliced thinly

- 1 cup canned artichokes

- 1 large cucumber, halved lengthwise and thinly sliced

- 5 ounces cream cheese, crumbled

Dressing

- ¼ cup extra-virgin olive oil

- 2 splashes white wine vinegar

- Coarse salt and black pepper

Directions:

Combine all of the dressing ingredients. Toss with the rest of the ingredients and combine well.

Peaches Cherries and Black Grape Salad

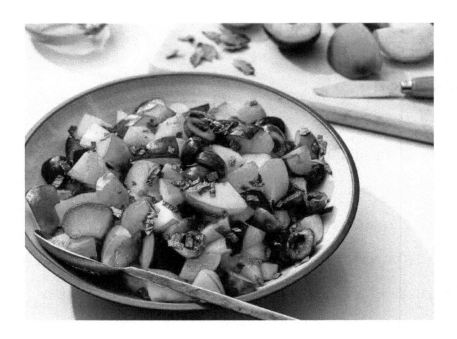

Ingredients:

- 1 cup of cubed peaches

- 1/4 cup cherries

- 12 pcs. black grapes

- 1/4 white onion, peeled, halved lengthwise, and thinly sliced

- 1 large cucumber, halved lengthwise and thinly sliced

- 5 ounces gouda cheese, shredded

<u>Dressing</u>

¼ cup extra-virgin olive oil

2 tbsp. apple cider vinegar

Coarse salt and black pepper

Directions:

Combine all of the dressing ingredients. Toss with the rest of the ingredients and combine well.

Kale Spinach and Watercress Salad

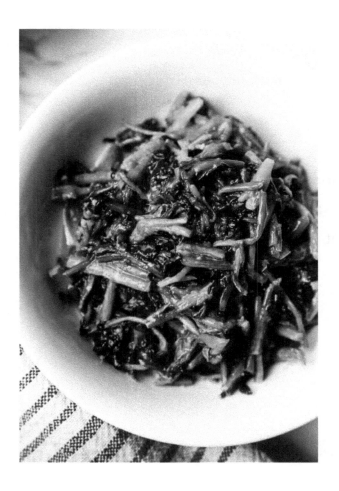

Ingredients:

- 1 bunch of kale, rinsed and drained

- 1 bunch of spinach, rinsed and drained

- 1 bunch of watercress, rinsed and drained

<u>Dressing</u>

- ¼ cup extra-virgin olive oil

- 2 splashes white wine vinegar

- Coarse salt and black pepper

Directions:

Combine all of the dressing ingredients. Toss with the rest of the ingredients and combine well.

Tomatoes Apples and Camambert Cheese Salad

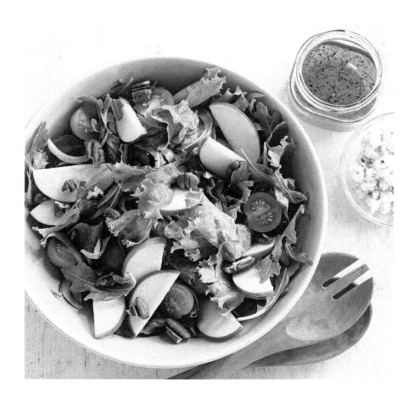

Ingredients:

- 5 medium tomatoes, halved lengthwise, seeded, and thinly sliced

- 1 cup Fuji apples cubed

- 1 cup of cubed peaches

- 1/4 cup cherries

- 5 ounces camembert cheese, crumbled

Dressing

- ¼ cup extra-virgin olive oil

- 2 splashes white wine vinegar

- Coarse salt and black pepper

Directions:

Combine all of the dressing ingredients. Toss with the rest of the ingredients and combine well

Apple Peaches and Cottage Cheese Salad

Ingredients:

- 10 Tomatillos, halved lengthwise, seeded, and thinly sliced
- 1 cup Fuji apples cubed
- 1 cup of cubed peaches
- 5 ounces cottage cheese, crumbled

<u>Dressing</u>

- ¼ cup extra-virgin olive oil
- 2 tbsp. apple cider vinegar
- Coarse salt and black pepper

Directions:

Combine all of the dressing ingredients. Toss with the rest of the ingredients and combine well.

Artichoke Red Cabbage and Parmesan Cheese Salad

Ingredients:

- 1/2 medium red cabbage, sliced thinly
- 1 cup canned artichokes
- 1 large cucumber, halved lengthwise and thinly sliced
- 5 ounces parmesan cheese, shredded

Dressing

- ¼ cup extra-virgin olive oil
- 2 splashes white wine vinegar
- Coarse salt and black pepper

Directions:

Combine all of the dressing ingredients. Toss with the rest of the ingredients and combine well.

Artichoke Napa Cabbage and Brie Cheese Salad

Ingredients:

- 1 cup canned artichokes
- 1/2 medium Napa cabbage, sliced thinly
- 1 large cucumber, halved lengthwise and thinly sliced
- 5 ounces brie cheese, crumbled

<u>Dressing</u>

- ¼ cup extra-virgin olive oil
- 2 splashes white wine vinegar
- Coarse salt and black pepper

Directions:

Combine all of the dressing ingredients. Toss with the rest of the ingredients and combine well.

Napa Cabbage Carrots and Parmesan Cheese Salad

Ingredients:

- 1/2 medium Napa cabbage, sliced thinly

- 5 baby carrots

- 5 ounces parmesan cheese, shredded

Dressing

- ¼ cup extra-virgin olive oil

- 2 tbsp. apple cider vinegar

- Coarse salt and black pepper

Directions:

Combine all of the dressing ingredients. Toss with the rest of the ingredients and combine well.

Watercress Spinach and Ricotta Salad

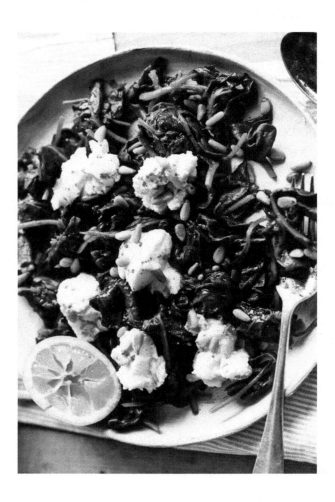

Ingredients:

- 10 Tomatillos, halved lengthwise, seeded, and thinly sliced

- 1 bunch of spinach, rinsed and drained

- 1 bunch of watercress, rinsed and drained

- 5 ounces ricotta cheese

Dressing

- ¼ cup extra-virgin olive oil

- 2 splashes white wine vinegar

- Coarse salt and black pepper

Directions:

Combine all of the dressing ingredients. Toss with the rest of the ingredients and combine well.

Spinach Peach and Pecorino Romano Salad

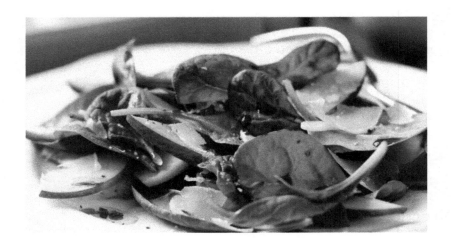

Ingredients:

- 1 bunch of Spinach, rinsed and drained

- 1 cup canned pineapple bits

- 1 cup of cubed peaches

- 5 ounces pecorino romano cheese, shredded

Dressing

- ¼ cup extra-virgin olive oil

- 2 splashes white wine vinegar

- Coarse salt and black pepper

Directions:

Combine all of the dressing ingredients. Toss with the rest of the ingredients and combine well.

Enoki Mushroom Red Cabbage and Monterey Jack Cheese Salad

Ingredients:

- 15 Enoki Mushrooms, thoroughly rinsed and thinly sliced
- 1/2 medium Red cabbage, sliced thinly
- 5 baby carrots
- 1 bunch of watercress, rinsed and drained
- 5 ounces monterey jack cheese, shredded

Dressing

1. ¼ cup extra-virgin olive oil
2. 2 splashes white wine vinegar
3. Coarse salt and black pepper

Directions:

Combine all of the dressing ingredients. Toss with the rest of the ingredients and combine well.

Napa Cabbage Artichokes and Parmesan Salad

Ingredients:

- 1 cup canned artichokes
- 1/2 medium Napa cabbage, sliced thinly
- 1/4 white onion, peeled, halved lengthwise, and thinly sliced
- 5 ounces parmesan cheese, shredded

Dressing

- ¼ cup extra-virgin olive oil
- 2 tbsp. apple cider vinegar
- Coarse salt and black pepper

Directions:

Combine all of the dressing ingredients. Toss with the rest of the ingredients and combine well.

Grape Corn and Feta Cheese Salad

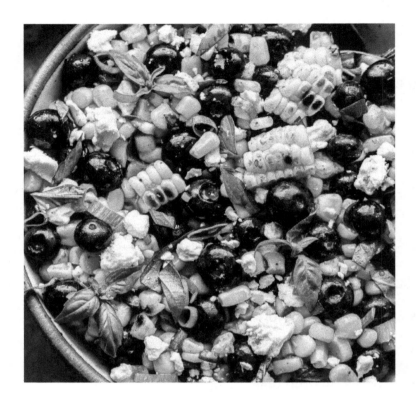

Ingredients:

- 1/2 cup pickles

- 10 pcs. red grapes

- 2 ounces feta cheese, crumbled

- 2 ounces pepperjack cheese, shredded

- 1 large cucumber, halved lengthwise and thinly sliced

- <u>Dressing</u>

  ¼ cup extra-virgin olive oil

- 2 splashes white wine vinegar

- Coarse salt and black pepper

Directions:

Combine all of the dressing ingredients. Toss with the rest of the ingredients and combine well.

Red Cabbage Apples and Ricotta Cheese Salad

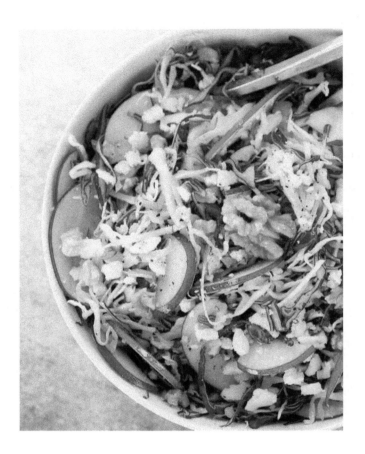

Ingredients:

- 1 cup Fuji apples cubed

- 1/2 medium red cabbage, sliced thinly

- 1/4 cup cherries

- 5 ounces ricotta cheese

- 1 large cucumber, halved lengthwise and thinly sliced

Dressing

- ¼ cup extra-virgin olive oil

- 2 splashes white wine vinegar

- Coarse salt and black pepper

Directions:

Combine all of the dressing ingredients. Toss with the rest of the ingredients and combine well

.

Plum Tomato Kale Pineapple and Feta Cheese Salad

Ingredients:

- 5 medium plum tomatoes, halved lengthwise, seeded, and thinly sliced
  1 bunch of kale, rinsed and drained
- 5 ounces feta cheese, crumbled
- 1 cup canned pineapple bits
- 1 cup of cubed mangoes

Dressing

- ¼ cup extra-virgin olive oil
- 2 splashes white wine vinegar
- Coarse salt and black pepper

Prep

Directions:

Combine all of the dressing ingredients. Toss with the rest of the ingredients and combine well.

Mango Tomatillo and Monterey Jack Cheese Salad

Ingredients:

- 10 Tomatillos, halved lengthwise, seeded, and thinly sliced
- 5 ounces monterey jack cheese, shredded
- 1 cup Fuji apples cubed
- 1/2 medium red cabbage, sliced thinly
- <u>Dressing</u>
  ¼ cup extra-virgin olive oil
- 2 tbsp. apple cider vinegar
- Coarse salt and black pepper

Directions:

Combine all of the dressing ingredients. Toss with the rest of the ingredients and combine well.

Broccoli Onion and Vegan Cheese Salad

Ingredients:

- 1 head broccoli florets and stems, blanched and cut into bite size pieces.

- 1/2 cup chopped white onion

- 1/2 cup raisins, optional

- 8 ounces vegan cheese, cut into very small chunks

- 1 cup egg-free mayonnaise

- 2 tablespoons red wine vinegar

- 1/4 cup honey

- 1/2 cup cherry tomatoes, halved

- Salt

- Freshly ground black pepper

Prep

Directions:

Toss all of the ingredients and combine well. Add more salt if necessary.

Simple Guacamole Salad

Ingredients:

- 1 pint cherry tomatoes, halved
- 1 green bell pepper, seeded and 1/2-inch diced
- 5 ounces feta cheese, crumbled
- 1/2 cup small diced red onion
- 2 tablespoons minced jalapeno peppers, seeded (2 peppers)
- 1/2 teaspoon freshly grated lemon zest
- 2 ripe avocados, seeded, peeled, and 1/2-inch diced

Dressing

- 1/4 cup freshly squeezed lemon juice
- 1/4 cup good olive oil
- 1 teaspoon kosher salt
- 1/2 teaspoon
- Freshly ground black pepper
- ¼ tsp. garlic powder
- 1/4 teaspoon ground cayenne pepper

Directions:

Combine all of the dressing ingredients. Toss with the rest of the ingredients and combine well.

Cherry Tomato and Monterey Jack Cheese Salad

Ingredients:

- 1 head broccoli florets and stems, blanched and cut into bite-sized pieces.

- 1/2 cup chopped white onion

- 1 ounce monterey jack cheese, shredded

- 2 ounces cheddar cheese , shredded

- 2 ounces pecorino romano cheese, shredded

- 8 ounces vegan cheese slices, sliced into thin strips

- 1/2 cup halved cherry tomatoes

Dressing

- 1 cup mayonnaise

- 2 tablespoons white wine vinegar

- 1/4 cup sugar

- Salt and freshly ground black pepper

Directions:

Combine all of the dressing ingredients. Toss with the rest of the ingredients and combine well.

Kidney Beans and Tomato Salad

Ingredients:

- 2 cans red kidney beans, drained, about 30 ounces
- 1 (15-ounce) can corn, drained
- 2 Roma tomatoes, diced
- 1/4 cup diced green bell pepper
- 1/4 cup diced red onion
- 1/4 cup diced green onions
- 1/4 cup diced pineapple
- 1 tablespoon chopped cilantro leaves
- 1 jalapeno, seeded and minced
- 4 tablespoons white wine vinegar
- Juice of ¼ lemon
- 3 tablespoons honey
- 1 tablespoons salt
- 1 teaspoon black pepper
- Pinch ground cumin

Directions:

Prep Combine all of the dressing ingredients. Toss all of the ingredients and combine well

Minimalist Roasted Tomatoes

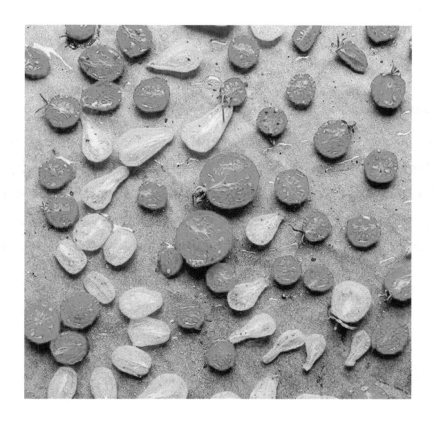

Ingredients:

- 30 ripe tomatoes, sliced in half crosswise.

- ¾ cup extra virgin olive oil

- 3 tbsp. Italian Seasoning

- 2 tbsp. Sea Salt

- ¼ cup Brown Sugar

- 2 ounces cheddar cheese, shredded

Directions:

Prep Preheat the oven to 170 degrees F. Place the tomatoes in a baking pan with the cut side up. Drizzle with 2/3 cup extra virgin olive oil, sugar, Italian seasoning and salt. Cook Bake for 10 hours. Drizzle with the remaining olive oil when you serve. Cook's Note: Do this overnight. You can use the roasted tomatoes to flavor almost any salad that you can imagine.

Minimalist Peach Mango and Cream Cheese Salad

Ingredients:

- 1 tbsp. ginger, minced
- Juice of 2 oranges
- 2 tsp. maple syrup
- ½ cup peaches, pitted and sliced
- 2 large mangoes, peeled and diced
- 2 ounces cream cheese, crumbled

Directions:

Mix the ginger and maple syrup with the Orange. juice. Toss the fruits with this mixture.

Grilled Eggplant and Pepperjack Cheese Salad

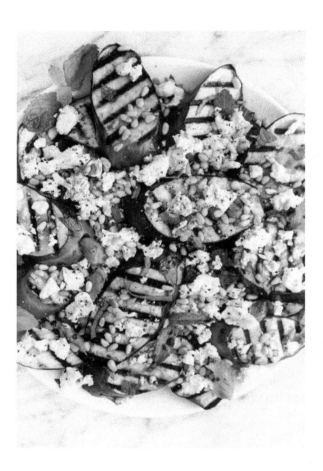

Ingredients:

- 30 ounces eggplant (about 12 ounces total), sliced lengthwise into 1/2-inch-thick rectangles

- ¼ cup macadamia nut oil

- 2 ounces pepperjack cheese, shredded

Dressing

- 2 tbsp. macadamia nut oil

- Steak seasoning, McCormick

- 3 tbsp. dry sherry

- 1 tbsp. dried thyme

Directions:

Preheat the grill to medium high. Brush the vegetables with ¼ cup oil. Cook Sprinkle with salt and pepper and grill for 4 min. per side. Flip once only so you can get the grill marks on the vegetable. Combine all of the dressing ingredients. Drizzle over the vegetable.

Grilled Zucchini and Asparagus Salad

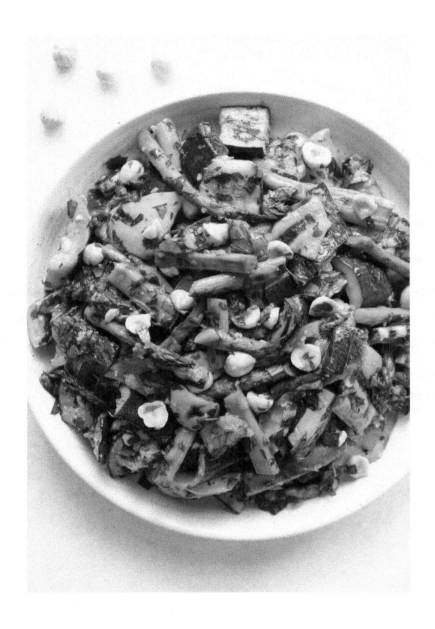

Ingredients:

- ¼ cup macadamia nut oil

- 1 pcs. Zucchini, cut lengthwise and cut in half

- 6 pcs. Asparagus

- 10 Cauliflower florets

- 5 pcs. Brussel Sprouts

- 2 ounces camembert cheese, crumbled

Dressing Ingredients

- 6 tbsp. olive oil

  3 dashes of Tabasco hot sauce

- Sea salt, to taste

- 3 tbsp. white wine vinegar

- 1 tsp. Egg-free mayonnaise

Prep

Directions:

Preheat the grill to medium high. Brush the vegetables with ¼ cup oil.

Cook Sprinkle with salt and pepper and grill for 4 min. per side. Flip once only so you can get the grill marks on the vegetable. Combine all of the dressing ingredients. Drizzle over the vegetable.

Grilled Cauliflower Brussel Sprout and Gouda Cheese Salad

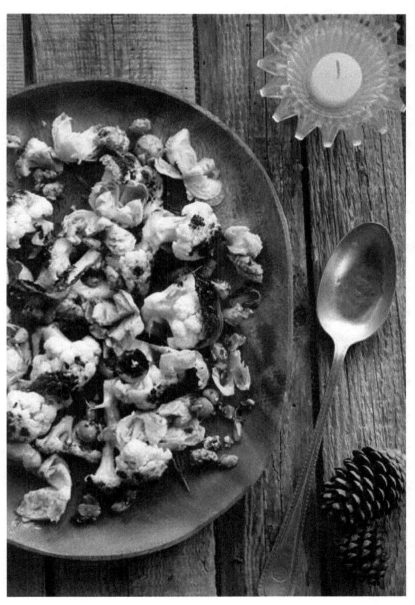

Ingredients:

- 5 Cauliflower florets
- 5 pcs. Brussel Sprouts
- 12 ounces eggplant, sliced lengthwise into 1/2-inch-thick rectangles
- 4 large Tomatoes, sliced thick
- 5 Cauliflower florets
- ¼ cup macadamia nut oil
- 2 ounces gouda cheese, shredded

<u>Dressing Ingredients</u>

- 4 tbsp. olive oil
- Steak seasoning, McCormick
- 2 tbsp. white vinegar
- 1 tbsp. dried thyme
- 1/2 tsp. sea salt

<u>Prep</u>

Directions:

Preheat the grill to medium high. Brush the vegetable with ¼ cup oil. Cook Sprinkle with salt and pepper and grill for 4 min. per side. Flip once only so you can get the grill marks on the vegetable. Combine all of the dressing ingredients. Drizzle over the vegetable.

Grilled Asparagus Eggplant and Ricotta Salad

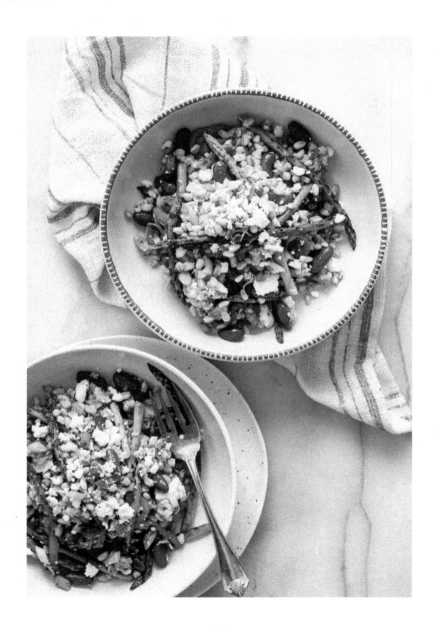

Ingredients:

- 1 pcs. Zucchini, cut lengthwise and cut in half

- 6 pcs. Asparagus

- 4 large Tomatoes, sliced thick

- 5 Cauliflower florets

- 30 ounces eggplant (about 12 ounces total), sliced lengthwise into 1/2-inch-thick rectangles

- ¼ cup extra virgin olive oil

- 2 ounces ricotta cheese

Dressing Ingredients

- 6 tbsp. olive oil

- 3 dashes of Tabasco hot sauce

- Sea salt, to taste

- 3 tbsp. white wine vinegar

- 1 tsp. Egg-free mayonnaise

Prep

Directions:

Preheat the grill to medium high. Brush the vegetable with ¼ cup oil. Cook Sprinkle with salt and pepper and grill for 4 min. per side. Flip once only so you can get the grill marks on the vegetable. Combine all of the dressing ingredients. Drizzle over the vegetable.

Grilled Eggplant Tomato and Pepperjack Cheese Salad

Ingredients:

- 10 ounces eggplant (about 12 ounces total), sliced lengthwise into 1/2-inch-thick rectangles

- 4 large Tomatoes, sliced thick

- 1 bunch endives

- 1/4 cup extra virgin olive oil

- 2 ounces pepperjack cheese, shredded

<u>Dressing Ingredients</u>

- 6 tbsp. extra virgin olive oil

- Sea salt, to taste

- 3 tbsp. apple cider vinegar

- 1 tbsp. honey

- 1 tsp. Egg-free mayonnaise

<u>Prep</u>

Directions:

Preheat the grill to medium high. Brush the vegetable with ¼ cup oil. Cook Sprinkle with salt and pepper and grill for 4 min. per side. Flip once only so you can get the grill marks on the vegetable. Combine all of the dressing ingredients. Drizzle over the vegetable.

Grilled Cauliflower Eggplant and Pecorino Romano Salad

Ingredients:

- 10 ounces eggplant (about 12 ounces total), sliced lengthwise into 1/2-inch-thick rectangles

- 5 Cauliflower florets

- 5 pcs. Brussel Sprouts

- ¼ cup extra virgin olive oil

- 2 ounces pecorino romano cheese, shredded

Dressing Ingredients

- 6 tbsp. olive oil

- 3 dashes of Tabasco hot sauce

- Sea salt, to taste

- 3 tbsp. white wine vinegar

- 1 tsp. Egg-free mayonnaise

Prep

Directions:

Preheat the grill to medium high. Brush the vegetable with ¼ cup oil. Cook Sprinkle with salt and pepper and grill for 4 min. per side. Flip once only so you can get the grill marks on the vegetable. Combine all of the dressing ingredients. Drizzle over the vegetable.

Grilled Green Beans Broccoli and Parmesan Salad 8 pcs.

Ingredients:

- 7 Broccoli florets

- 9 ounces eggplant (about 12 ounces total), sliced lengthwise into 1/2-inch-thick rectangles

- 1 bunch endives

- 1/4 cup extra virgin olive oil

- 2 ounces parmesan cheese, shredded

Dressing Ingredients

- 6 tbsp. extra virgin olive oil

- Sea salt, to taste

- 3 tbsp. apple cider vinegar

- 1 tbsp. honey

- 1 tsp. Egg-free mayonnaise

Prep

Directions:

Preheat the grill to medium high. Brush the vegetable with ¼ cup oil. Cook Sprinkle with salt and pepper and grill for 4 min. per side. Flip once only so you can get the grill marks on the vegetable. Combine all of the dressing ingredients. Drizzle over the vegetable.

Grilled Green Beans Broccoli and Feta Cheese Salad

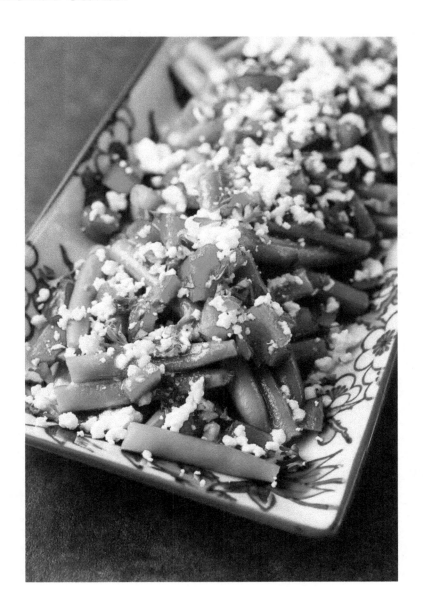

Ingredients:

- 8 pcs. Green Beans
- 7 Broccoli florets 10 ounces eggplant (about 12 ounces total), sliced lengthwise into 1/2-inch-thick rectangles
- 1 pcs. Zucchini, cut lengthwise and cut in half
- 6 pcs. Asparagus
- ¼ cup extra virgin olive oil
- 2 ounces feta cheese, crumbled

Dressing Ingredients

- 6 tbsp. olive oil
- 3 dashes of Tabasco hot sauce
- Sea salt, to taste
- 3 tbsp. white wine vinegar
- 1 tsp. Egg-free mayonnaise

Prep

Directions:

Preheat the grill to medium high. Brush the vegetable with ¼ cup oil. Cook Sprinkle with salt and pepper and grill for 4 min. per side. Flip once only so you can get the grill marks on the vegetable. Combine all of the dressing ingredients. Drizzle over the vegetable.

Grilled Cauliflower Brussel Sprout and Mozarella Cheese Salad

Ingredients:

- 5 Cauliflower florets

- 5 pcs. Brussel Sprouts

- 30 ounces eggplant (about 12 ounces total), sliced lengthwise into 1/2-inch-thick rectangles

- ¼ cup extra virgin olive oil

- 2 ounces mozarella cheese, shredded

<u>Dressing Ingredients</u>

- 6 tbsp. extra virgin olive oil

- Sea salt, to taste

- 3 tbsp. apple cider vinegar

- 1 tbsp. honey

- 1 tsp. Egg-free mayonnaise

<u>Prep</u>

Directions:

Preheat the grill to medium high. Brush the vegetable with ¼ cup oil. Cook Sprinkle with salt and pepper and grill for 4 min. per side. Flip once only so you can get the grill marks on the vegetable. Combine all of the dressing ingredients. Drizzle over the vegetable.

Grilled Green Beans and Tomato Salad

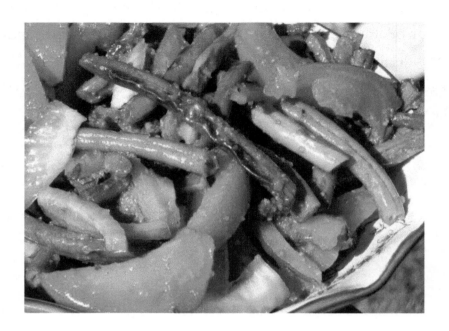

Ingredients:

- 8 pcs. Green Beans

- 7 Broccoli florets

- 4 large Tomatoes, sliced thick

- 5 Cauliflower florets

- ¼ cup macadamia nut oil

Dressing Ingredients

- 4 tbsp. olive oil

- Steak seasoning, McCormick

- 2 tbsp. white vinegar

- 1 tbsp. dried thyme

- 1/2 tsp. sea salt

Prep

Directions:

Preheat the grill to medium high. Brush the vegetable with ¼ cup oil. Cook Sprinkle with salt and pepper and grill for 4 min. per side. Flip once only so you can get the grill marks on the vegetable. Combine all of the dressing ingredients. Drizzle over the vegetable.

Spicy Grilled Eggplant Endives Salad

Ingredients:

- 10 ounces eggplant (about 12 ounces total), sliced
- lengthwise into 1/2-inch-thick rectangles
- 1 bunch endives
- 1/4 cup extra virgin olive oil

<u>Dressing Ingredients</u>

- 6 tbsp. olive oil
- 3 dashes of Tabasco hot sauce
- Sea salt, to taste
- 3 tbsp. white wine vinegar
- 1 tsp. Egg-free mayonnaise

<u>Prep</u>

Directions:

Preheat the grill to medium high. Brush the vegetable with ¼ cup oil. Cook Sprinkle with salt and pepper and grill for 4 min. per side. Flip once only so you can get the grill marks on the vegetable. Combine all of the dressing ingredients. Drizzle over the vegetable.

Grilled Cauliflower Brussel Sprout and Cheddar Salad

Ingredients:

- 5 Cauliflower florets

- 5 pcs. Brussel Sprouts

- 1 ounce monterey jack cheese, shredded

- 2 ounces cheddar cheese, shredded

Dressing Ingredients

- 6 tbsp. extra virgin olive oil

- Sea salt, to taste

- 3 tbsp. apple cider vinegar

- 1 tbsp. honey

- 1 tsp. Egg-free mayonnaise

Prep

Directions:

Preheat the grill to medium high. Brush the vegetable with ¼ cup oil. Cook Sprinkle with salt and pepper and grill for 4 min.

84

per side. Flip once only so you can get the grill marks on the vegetable. Combine all of the dressing ingredients. Drizzle over the vegetable.

Grilled Asparagus and Cheese Salad

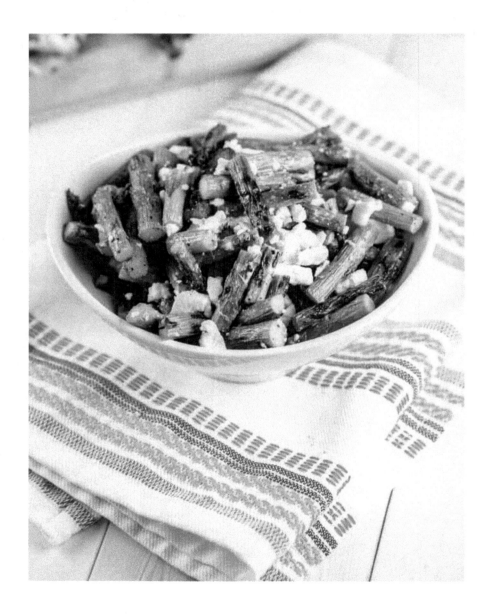

Ingredients:

- 1 pcs. Zucchini, cut lengthwise and cut in half

- 6 pcs. Asparagus

- 30 ounces eggplant (about 12 ounces total), sliced lengthwise into 1/2-inch-thick rectangles

- 2 ounces cheddar cheese, shredded

- 2 ounces pecorino romano cheese, shredded

Dressing Ingredients

- 6 tbsp. olive oil

- 3 dashes of Tabasco hot sauce

- Sea salt, to taste

- 3 tbsp. white wine vinegar

- 1 tsp. Egg-free mayonnaise

Prep

Directions:

Preheat the grill to medium high. Brush the vegetable with ¼ cup oil.

Cook Sprinkle with salt and pepper and grill for 4 min. per side. Flip once only so you can get the grill marks on the vegetable. Combine all of the dressing ingredients. Drizzle over the vegetable.

Grilled Zucchini Asparagus & Gouda Cheese Salad

Ingredients:

- 10 ounces eggplant (about 12 ounces total), sliced lengthwise into 1/2-inch-thick rectangles

- 1 pcs. Zucchini, cut lengthwise and cut in half

- 6 pcs. Asparagus

- 2 ounces brie cheese, crumbled

- 2 ounces gouda cheese, shredded

Dressing Ingredients

- 4 tbsp. olive oil

- Steak seasoning, McCormick

- 2 tbsp. white vinegar

- 1 tbsp. dried thyme

- 1/2 tsp. sea salt

Prep

Directions:

Preheat the grill to medium high. Brush the vegetable with ¼ cup oil. Cook Sprinkle with salt and pepper and grill for 4 min. per side. Flip once only so you can get the grill marks on the vegetable. Combine all of the dressing ingredients. Drizzle over the vegetable.

Grilled Endives Green Bean and Ricotta Cheese Salad

Ingredients:

- 5 Cauliflower florets

- 5 pcs. Brussel Sprouts

- 8 pcs. Green Beans

- 7 Broccoli florets

- 1 bunch endives

- 2 ounces parmesan cheese, shredded

- 2 ounces ricotta cheese

Dressing Ingredients

- 6 tbsp. extra virgin olive oil

- Sea salt, to taste

- 3 tbsp. apple cider vinegar

- 1 tbsp. honey

- 1 tsp. Egg-free mayonnaise

Directions:

Prep Preheat the grill to medium high. Brush the vegetable with ¼ cup oil. Cook Sprinkle with salt and pepper and grill for 4 min. per side. Flip once only so you can get the grill marks on the vegetable. Combine all of the dressing ingredients. Drizzle over the vegetable.

Grilled Eggplant Zucchini and Feta Cheese Salad

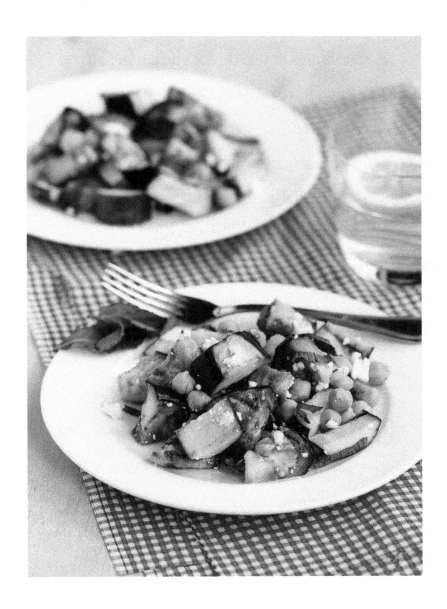

Ingredients:

- 10 ounces eggplant (about 12 ounces total), sliced lengthwise into 1/2-inch-thick rectangles
- 1 pcs. Zucchini, cut lengthwise and cut in half
- 4 large Tomatoes, sliced thick
- 1 bunch endives
- 1/4 cup extra virgin olive oil
- 2 ounces feta cheese, crumbled
- 2 ounces pepperjack cheese, shredded

Dressing

- 2 tbsp. macadamia nut oil
- Steak seasoning, McCormick
- 3 tbsp. dry sherry
- 1 tbsp. dried thyme

Prep

Directions:

Preheat the grill to medium high. Brush the vegetable with ¼ cup oil. Cook Sprinkle with salt and pepper and grill for 4 min. per side. Flip once only so you can get the grill marks on the vegetable. Combine all of the dressing ingredients. Drizzle over the vegetable.

Grilled Asparagus Zucchini and Ricotta Cheese Salad

Ingredients:

- 2 ounces camembert cheese, crumbled

- 2 ounces parmesan cheese, shredded

- 2 ounces ricotta cheese

- 6 pcs. Asparagus spears

- 12 ounces eggplant (about 12 ounces total), sliced lengthwise into 1/2-inch-thick rectangles

- ¼ cup extra virgin olive oil

<u>Dressing Ingredients</u>

- 6 tbsp. olive oil

- 3 dashes of Tabasco hot sauce

- Sea salt, to taste

- 3 tbsp. white wine vinegar

- 1 tsp. Egg-free mayonnaise

<u>Prep</u>

Directions:

Preheat the grill to medium high. Brush the vegetable with ¼ cup oil. Cook Sprinkle with salt and pepper and grill for 4 min. per side. Flip once only so you can get the grill marks on the vegetable. Combine all of the dressing ingredients. Drizzle over the vegetable.

Grilled Mango Apple and Brussel Sprouts Salad

Ingredients:

- 1 cup of cubed mangoes

- 1 cup Fuji apples cubed

- 5 pcs. Brussel Sprouts

- ¼ cup extra virgin olive oil

Dressing Ingredients

- 6 tbsp. extra virgin olive oil

- Sea salt, to taste

- 3 tbsp. apple cider vinegar

- 1 tbsp. honey

- 1 tsp. Egg-free mayonnaise

Prep

Directions:

Preheat the grill to medium high. Brush the vegetable with ¼ cup oil. Cook Sprinkle with salt and pepper and grill for 4 min. per side. Flip once only so you can get the grill marks on the vegetable. Combine all of the dressing ingredients. Drizzle over the vegetable.

Grilled Kale Eggplant and Blue Cheese Salad

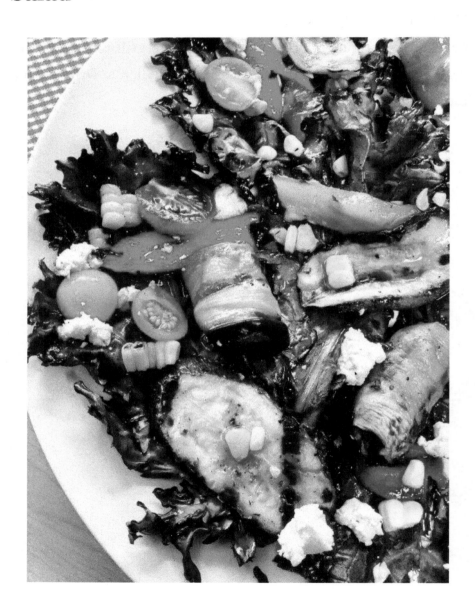

Ingredients:

- 12 ounces eggplant (about 12 ounces total), sliced lengthwise into 1/2-inch-thick rectangles
- 1 bunch of kale, rinsed and drained
- 1 cup canned pineapple bits
- 2 ounces gouda cheese, shredded
- 2 ounce blue cheese, crumbled

Dressing

- 2 tbsp. macadamia nut oil
- Steak seasoning, McCormick
- 3 tbsp. dry sherry
- 1 tbsp. dried thyme

Prep

Directions:

Preheat the grill to medium high. Brush the vegetable with ¼ cup oil.

Cook Sprinkle with salt and pepper and grill for 4 min. per side. Flip once only so you can get the grill marks on the vegetable. Combine all of the dressing ingredients. Drizzle over the vegetable.

Grilled Kale Green Bean and Mozzarella Cheese Salad

Ingredients:

- 8 pcs. Green Beans

- 1 bunch of kale, rinsed and drained

- 2 ounces feta cheese, crumbled

- 2 ounces mozarella cheese, shredded

Dressing

- 2 tbsp. macadamia nut oil

- Steak seasoning, McCormick

- 3 tbsp. dry sherry

- 1 tbsp. dried thyme

Prep

Directions:

Preheat the grill to medium high. Brush the vegetable with ¼ cup oil. Cook Sprinkle with salt and pepper and grill for 4 min.

per side. Flip once only so you can get the grill marks on the vegetable. Combine all of the dressing ingredients. Drizzle over the vegetable.

Grilled Carrots Watercress and Cottage Cheese Salad

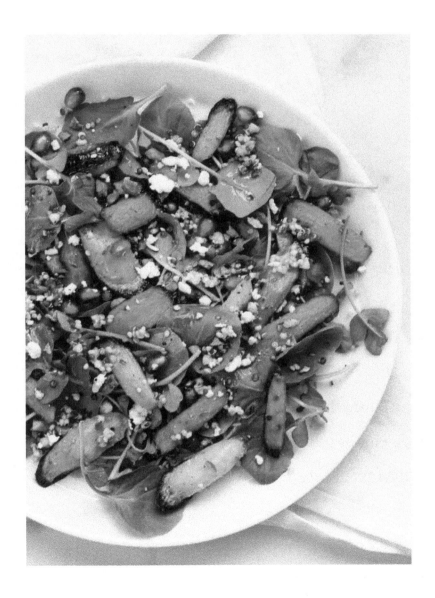

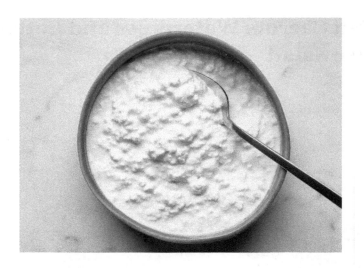

Ingredients:

- 12 ounces eggplant (about 12 ounces total), sliced lengthwise into 1/2-inch-thick rectangles

- 5 baby carrots

- 1 bunch of watercress, rinsed and drained

- 1 bunch endives

- 2 ounces brie cheese, crumbled

- 2 ounces cottage cheese, crumbled

Dressing Ingredients

- 6 tbsp. olive oil

- 3 dashes of Tabasco hot sauce

- Sea salt, to taste

- 3 tbsp. white wine vinegar

- 1 tsp. Egg-free mayonnaise

<u>Prep</u>

Directions:

Preheat the grill to medium high. Brush the vegetable with ¼ cup oil. Cook Sprinkle with salt and pepper and grill for 4 min. per side. Flip once only so you can get the grill marks on the vegetable. Combine all of the dressing ingredients. Drizzle over the vegetable.